Great Sex!. Over Size: An Uncensored Sex Secrets Guide to Amazing, Exciting, and Sensational Sex Techniques that will Make Her Happy Irrespective of Size

By

Patti W. Nieves

Copyright Statement:

Disclaimer:

The information provided in "Great Sex! Over Size: An Uncensored Sex Secrets Guide to Amazing, Exciting, and Sensational Sex Techniques that will Make Her Happy Irrespective of Size" is intended for educational and entertainment purposes only. The author, Patti W. Nieves, is not a licensed therapist, medical professional, or certified sexologist.

Readers are encouraged to consult with qualified healthcare professionals for personalized advice regarding their individual situations. The author and publisher disclaim any liability for any adverse effects resulting directly or indirectly from the use or application of the information contained in this book.

The techniques, advice, and suggestions presented in this guide are based on the author's research, personal experiences, and interviews with experts in the field. It is essential for readers to exercise their discretion and judgment in applying any recommendations to their own circumstances.

This guide may contain explicit content and discussions related to intimate relationships. Readers are advised that individual experiences may vary, and the author does not endorse or encourage any behavior that goes against legal or ethical standards.

By engaging with this guide, readers acknowledge and agree to the terms of this disclaimer. The author and publisher are not responsible for any consequences resulting from the use of the information provided in this publication.

About the Author: Patti W. Nieves

Patti W. Nieves, the creative mind behind "Great Sex! Over Size," is a passionate content creator at the forefront of the movement for sexual satisfaction. With a profound commitment to reshaping narratives around intimacy, Patti brings a wealth of knowledge and a fresh perspective to the exploration of pleasure beyond societal norms.

Patti's journey into the realm of sexual wellness and satisfaction began with a dedication to understanding the intricacies of human desire and connection. As a content creator, Patti has been a driving force in dismantling stereotypes and fostering an environment where individuals can embrace their unique desires without judgment.

Having curated a diverse range of content that navigates the complexities of intimacy, Patti is recognized for her uncensored approach to sex education. With a focus on empowering individuals to prioritize techniques over size, Patti has become a trusted guide for those seeking to enhance their intimate relationships.

Through a blend of insightful research, candid discussions, and a commitment to inclusivity, Patti

W. Nieves has established herself as a leading voice in the conversation about sexual satisfaction. "Great Sex! Over Size" is a testament to her dedication to providing a comprehensive, uncensored guide that invites readers to explore the depths of pleasure and prioritize the artistry of intimacy.

As you embark on this journey guided by Patti's expertise, you'll find a refreshing and empowering perspective on sex, where satisfaction is not confined by societal expectations. Get ready to uncover amazing, exciting, and sensational sex techniques that will make her happy, irrespective of size, under the thoughtful guidance of Patti W. Nieves – a trailblazer in the pursuit of sexual satisfaction for all.

Table of Content

Introduction

Navigating the Depths of Pleasure

Welcome to "Great Sex! Over Size," an uncensored manual that explores the world of incredible, thrilling, and sensational sex techniques by going beyond social conventions. This guide invites you on a trip beyond size restrictions, exploring the beauty of intimacy and the secrets that lead to true fulfillment in a world too frequently consumed with surface standards.

The experience of sexual pleasure is a complex and highly personal fabric that is stitched together by communication, wants, and technical proficiency. We dispel common misconceptions in this unedited exploration and provide you with the facts you need to establish a close bond that exceeds space and time. This book is your friend while you explore the mysteries of pleasure, whether your goal is to improve your relationship or start a new one.

Come along as we explore the fine distinction of intimacy and provide insight into methods that put an emphasis on communication, connection, and the celebration of a range of needs. This is more than simply a manual; it's an invitation to redefine and improve your perception of pleasure and pave the way for a rewarding and thrilling sexual experience. Let's explore this world of limitless pleasure and uninhibited secrets that lead the art form of satisfaction.

Common Misconceptions Regarding Size.

Men, like women, are obsessed with their bodies. Too small, too tall, or too fat And as we all know, a lot of people are particularly fixated with their gear. Many people worry about their penis' size and form, especially when it comes to their sexual compatibility with their spouse. But there's no one size fits all, and there are other significant aspects of compatibility besides penile size.

The size of the human penis varies greatly, and a significant percentage of adult males suffer from anxiety related to their body size.

Your partner's level of sexual enjoyment is not always determined by your penis' size. Many guys seem to be concerned about this variety, as many will try everything it takes to enlarge their penis, including taking pills, buying weight systems, vacuum pumps, stretching devices, silicone injections, or penis augmentation. Sexual compatibility is an essential component for many sexual partners.

Nonetheless, research indicates that penis size is not the primary determinant of sexual satisfaction.

There is a widespread belief in society that a person's sexual satisfaction or ability is mostly dependent on physical attributes like size.

These ideas regarding the role that size plays in sexual fulfillment are frequently based on misconceptions and preconceptions that do not accurately represent the variety of intimate relationship reality. Among these impressions are the following:

1. Size Equals Performance: It's a common misperception that greater physical size equates to improved sexual performance. This oversimplification misses the many other elements that go into having a great sexual encounter, including as technique, emotional connection, and communication.

2. Pressure to Conform to Norms: People are unfairly pressured to adhere to social norms that set forth particular standards for what constitutes a "ideal" size. This can undermine confidence and self-esteem by causing fears and feelings of inadequacy.

3. All-inclusive Expectations: It can be restrictive when society encourages a one-size-fits-all method

of achieving sexual fulfillment. Since each person and relationship are unique, what works for one may not necessarily work for another. This viewpoint downplays how important it is to recognize and accommodate each person's unique preferences and needs.

4. Stigmatization of Smaller Sizes: There is a propensity in society to link smaller sizes to a lower level of femininity or masculinity. This stigma may have an adverse effect on people's mental and emotional health by feeding unjustified expectations and damaging perceptions.

5. Silence and Lack of Conversation: A lack of fruitful conversation might result from societal unease with candid conversations regarding sexual issues. This silence could aid in the spread of false information about the complex issues and help to keep misconceptions alive.

Prioritizing action above tool size in sexual activities highlights the importance of involvement, skill, and entire experience instead of overemphasizing physical characteristics. This method acknowledges that an intimate relationship that is both full and rewarding involves a number of variables that go beyond physical dimensions.

To uncover the greatest sex advice we've ever offered, we combed through hundreds of Men's Health articles about relationships and sex. These suggestions are sourced from a variety of medical professionals, therapists, and specialists in the US who focus on intimacy, enjoyment, and sexual health.

Emphasis on the Importance of Sexual Actions and Techniques Over Size

Though not as much as to get her to the climax, penis size counts. Large penises may appeal to many women, but girth is more important than length. Women can benefit much from having a penis with the proper girth and size, and proper technique is obviously essential.

Guys with a little one and a very normal, thick girth. Any woman can climax thanks to the girth, even though the penis only extended five inches (when it was hard). You can compensate for your size by combining skillful maneuvers. If a man learns how to use his small penis, it's not awful at all.

In actuality, both size and technique matter, but technique is more important. Not even the biggest

dick in the world will get a lady to climax if you are
not skilled at making love to her.
Technique (foreplay and much more) is more
crucial than size, as evidenced by the fact that most
women do not climax from penetration. Also, penile
augmentation operations and condoms were
recommended if size was more essential than
technique.

Furthermore, regardless of size, a man's actions in
the bedroom or the quality of his sex with a woman
are primarily determined by his feelings for her and
his level of generosity or selfishness. Big dicks and
small dicks: orgasms are more often related to the
effort men put in to persuade their ladies to suck
than they are to the size and length of their little
man.

Technique is particularly important because some
women have extreme fetishes and want total
gratification from their partners in bed. In light of
this, technique matters and foreplay is essential.
Here, size might not be very important.

Just so you know, there's more than just a penis to
get a girl to cum!

Therefore, technique is more important than size in this situation. Guys shouldn't feel self-conscious about their size at all. It's concerning if they lose it in bed due to poor technique.

There's no skill without a tool and even the best of tools are useless without skill.

Chapter One: Dispelling Myths: Size is Not Everything

Anxiety about penis size is widespread. Nonetheless, the majority of persons who worry about the size or form of their penis typically fall within normal ranges. A person's partner may frequently be indifferent to their size. In some cases, anxiety rather than size may be the primary issue.

Concerns about whether their penis is large enough and will satisfy a sexual partner are common. A person's self-esteem and confidence may be impacted by this. But these worries are frequently unjustified.

Having sex can be more enjoyable if there is open communication, sex therapy support, and a willingness to try new things, regardless of the size or shape of either partner.

According to a 2020 study, the majority of men think that an erect penis typically measures 15.2 centimeters (cm) or 6 inches (in). The average is actually somewhat lower.

The average length is probably between 12.9 and 13.97 cm (5.1 and 5.5 in), with a large range of sizes; it is most likely on the lesser end of this scale. The majority of research estimate the average to be

within this range, while the results vary
significantly.
A micropenis, which is an abnormally small penis,
is a birth defect that is typically caused by hormonal
or genetic reasons. The functions of a micropenis
are the same as those of an average-sized penis, but
its look may not satisfy certain people. If a person
desires, surgery or hormone therapy can enlarge it.

A penis of ordinary size may appear smaller at
times due to extra skin surrounding it. This is
sometimes referred to as a "buried penis," and it
can be fixed surgically.
Research on penis size is still ongoing and yields
comparable results. Individual differences in penis
size can be attributed to a variety of factors,
including age, genetics, and general health.

Furthermore, the technique of measurement (e.g.,
self-reported versus measured by a healthcare
expert) can have an impact on the results. The idea
of what constitutes a "normal" penis size is
primarily culturally constructed and varies widely
among nations. One should not experience
insecurity or self-consciousness due to their penis
size. Research indicates that most women are OK
with the size of their partner's penis, and that
emotional closeness and communication have a

greater influence on sexual satisfaction than
physical appearance.
There is a fairly widespread misconception that
when it comes to sex, bigger is better. However,
research indicates that it is not at all like that. All of
it is mental! Because it's all in your head, your most
active organ for sex is your imagination.

Numerous examples exist where a man's little
stature can nonetheless elicit sexual pleasure from
women, dispelling the stereotype that size matters
not at all!

Women can have anxiety over size because it is
something that enters their body. They might enjoy
their sex life and feel at peace with a small one.

Most women, regardless of size, find it a little
challenging to experience an orgasm. The
important thing about sex is its quality. There are
various sex positions available, and men who feel
that their size is insufficient might experiment with
other approaches to make women feel good about
themselves. Women will remember his efforts to be
an incredible lover.

Not only do males experience it, but women also
struggle with their own size. The feeling of having a

large penis can be excruciating, painful, and first frightening for someone with a small vagina. Thus, in this instance, a little man emerges as the dazzling knight. They assist people in having nice, painless sex with lots of foreplay.

For millennia, people have argued and discussed penis size. There are still a lot of myths and misconceptions about penis size, even after a lot of studies and research has been done on the issue. To help dispel any uncertainty and offer clarification, we will look at some of the most prevalent myths and facts regarding penis size in this chapter.

1. Myth: Having a bigger penis is always preferable. Fact: The size of a penis does not determine a partner's level of sexual satisfaction or pleasure. Better sex is not a given, but having a larger penis can mean more physical stimulation. In fact, a partner may experience pain or discomfort occasionally due to a bigger penis.

2. Myth: Genetics determines the size of a flaccid penis
Fact: Although a penis's size when it is erect is mostly determined by heredity, a penis's size when it is flaccid or at rest can be influenced by a variety of other circumstances. These include temperature,

the time of day, general fitness, and hormone levels. One's actual penis size is not at all predicted by the size of their penis when at rest.

3. Myth: A small penis is unusual
Fact: An erect penis typically measures 5.16 inches in length. There is, nevertheless, a substantial variation in the normal penis size; some men have larger penises than others. It is natural and not cause for alarm that the penis is smaller.

4. Myth: Exercise and supplements can make your penis bigger.
Fact: There is no scientific proof to back up the claim that taking vitamins or exercising can make your penis get bigger. Many of these products actually have the potential to be dangerous and perhaps permanently damaging.

5. Myth: Your shoe or foot size determines your penis size.
Fact: There are distinct hereditary elements that influence a man's penis size and his feet size. The size of a person's bones, together with the quantity of fat and muscle tissue present, define the size of their feet. On the other hand, the quantity of blood flow and blood arteries in the region dictate the size of a man's penis. Furthermore, a man's shoe size

might differ significantly according on the type and brand of footwear.

The size of a man's penis is not a sign of his masculinity or how he feels about his sex. As each person is unique, there is no such thing as a "normal" penis size.

6. Myth: It is possible to lengthen or enlarge the penis.
Fact: Although surgical procedures can be used to cure anatomical abnormalities like phimosis and/or paraphimosis and Peyronie's disease, the penis cannot be made longer or larger. According to the American Urological Association, penile lengthening is a risky and inefficient surgery (AUA).

7. Myth: A small penis isn't ideal for intimate relations.
Fact: Extremely inflated expectations of sex and the parts needed to achieve it have been propagated by the entertainment industry and the media. It's important to always keep in mind that there is no perfect penis length or girth that results in the greatest sex. Yes, there are preferences, but all penis sizes are acceptable and capable of having satisfying sex.

8. Myth: The only thing that causes orgasms and enjoyable sex is a big penis.
Fact: The idea of having the "perfect penis" is quite intriguing, yet preferences are really personal. Not only can a "large penis" result in satisfying sex, but so can a smaller one. There is no clear correlation between size and satisfying sex, orgasms, or pleasure. Males frequently worry that their penis is "too small." A small penis, on the other hand, is actually less than 3 inches when erect; anything greater than 3 inches is considered normal. Although most people don't care about size, it is normal for males to feel anxious about this.

9. Myth: You can't get orgasms from a small penis
Fact: There is no relationship between a person's capacity for pleasure and orgasm and the size of their penis. The degree of stimulation during sex is, in fact, more crucial to reaching an orgasm than the size of the penis. The vaginal and penile regions are extremely sensitive to touch and are readily aroused by a variety of touch techniques, such as oral sex and manual stimulation.
To have an orgasm, emotional and psychological aspects are just as important as physical stimulation. A fulfilling sexual encounter is mostly dependent on having a cheerful and carefree attitude, communicating, and having faith in one's

partner. Each person is unique, and some may like certain types of stimulation over others. In order to figure out what works best for them, partners should talk to each other and try different things.

10. Myth: People find penises with increased size more attractive
Fact: It's a fallacy that a bigger penis makes a person look more handsome. Studies have indicated that there is minimal or no relationship between a man's and a woman's penis size and sexual satisfaction. Women are actually more concerned with other aspects of a partner, like as communication, emotional connection, and sexual technique, according to studies.

11. Myth: A penis that measures less than 6-7 inches is deemed "small."
This is a complete myth. A little penis, medically referred to as a Micropenis, is defined as one whose stretched penile length (SPL) is about less than 3 inches (7.62 cm). Anything that is stretched beyond 3 inches is regarded as normal.

12. Myth: The penis gets smaller with excessive masturbation
Fact: The corpora cavernosa refers to the outer two of the penis's three major chambers. During an

erection, blood fills these chambers, which are in charge of the penis's erectile function. There are many who think that overindulging in masturbation can cause these chambers to contract, resulting in a smaller penis. Nevertheless, this assertion is unsupported by any data. Genetics determines the size of the penis; sexual activity or inactivity has no bearing on it. Masturbation does not cause the penis to enlarge or contract.

It's also important to remember that masturbating is a normal and healthy aspect of sexuality in people. It can strengthen the immune system, lessen stress, and enhance sleep. There is no reason to refrain from masturbating as it does not pose any harm to the penis. In reality, research indicates that men who ejaculate frequently (by sexual activity or masturbation) are less likely to get prostate cancer.

There isn't a single "normal" penis size—everyone's body is unique. We urge you to appreciate and be aware of your physical attributes rather than putting undue focus on penis size or comparing yourself to other people. Recall that penis size is not a sign of masculinity or a predictor of sexual satisfaction or enjoyment for either partner.

Women's Sexual Pleasure and Penis Size

There are two aspects to the size problem as well: breadth (width) and length . However, most discussions of size refer to length. For this reason, the typical length of a man's organ in the United States is said to be between five and seven inches. In other regions and research, the length typically receives the most immediate attention. However, studies have indicated that women find greater pleasure in the male organ's width than in its length.

The fact that the vagina adjusts to accommodate the size of the male organ has led renowned sex researchers to further conclude that the size of the male organ cannot truly have a physiological impact on a woman's level of sexual enjoyment. It's flexible. Therefore, the researcher came to the conclusion that any size penis will fit and give a female appropriate sexual excitement, despite the concerns of many men over penis size.

Women's perceptions of the significance of penile size are subjective. There are a variety of elements that could influence how much value women place on penis size. Whether this is a physical or psychological phenomenon is unknown. Some

women who have been exposed to porn may think that having a big penis is normal or even attractive. According to certain theories, women may place less value on penis size in long-term relationships than they do on transient closeness.
Stretch receptors found in the vagina are partially in charge of a woman's feelings during intercourse. It is conceivable that a larger penis might produce more feeling during intimacy in women whose vaginal vaults are larger as a result of natural delivery.

When considering penile sizes from the standpoint of physical sensation, there could be a variety of acceptable sizes. Some women describe closeness and agony associated with huge penis sizes, while other women claim very small penis sizes causing them to lose feeling.
A possible explanation for sexual experience could be a mix of relative male and female body sizes. Thus far, this has not been the subject of any scientific inquiry.

Not Your Penis Size, But What Women Want in
Bed

1. Improved Communication: According to survey
data, around 62% of women stated that their
marriages would be enhanced by improved
communication. But they weren't by themselves. A
little over half of the guys polled concurred.
To have a fulfilling and passionate sexual life with
your spouse in any relationship, you both need to
be aware of each other's preferences. Even after
you've been dating for a while, discussing sex can
still feel a bit strange. Bring up your personal
desires to let her know you want to talk about them
if you want to start a conversation. Next, inform her
that you're prepared to provide whatever assistance
you can.

After that, tell her you'll do everything in your
power to give her the pleasure she desires. Just be
as sincere and honest as you can when bringing it
up in a casual setting, such as after dinner or while
you're out for a solo stroll.

2. More Foreplay: Since sex is about much more
than just having sex and getting high, it's hardly
surprising that 58% of women would be okay with
you emphasizing foreplay more.

Oral sex, kissing, and other actions that are
commonly regarded as foreplay are all components
of sexual activity. Orgasm and sexual activity are
the cherry on top.
Spending time to physically stimulate her will cause
her body to produce more lubricant in the vagina
which plays a big role in making sex more of and
comfortable for her.

To turn her on, you don't even have to be in bed:
Foreplay is defined as any action you take that
increases desire in her, such as sending her sultry
photographs and compliments, planning dinner for
her, and texting her throughout the day.

3. Sex toys: According to a survey of women, 40% of
them, sex toys are very beneficial in the bedroom.
Too often, men perceive the idea of sex toys as a
threat, believing it to be a reflection of their
masculinity or lack thereof. However, sex toys can
inject some innovation and fun into usually
mundane sex positions. For instance, utilizing a
smaller vibrator can provide her with more manual
stimulation in positions where her clitoris isn't able
to naturally rub against you, which is something
many women want in order to experience an
orgasm.

A vibrating penis ring should do the trick if you want to try something that will feel fantastic for both of you.

4. Fantasies: Although having sexual fantasies and fetishes is usually frowned upon, 40% of women said that giving in to them would improve their marriages. Furthermore, half of the men agreed with the concept.
Though it's not for everyone, living out a fantasy can develop into a close-knit bonding experience if you're open to trying new things.
Not all fantasies involve whippings and bondage. Sometimes it's just an indication that she wants to try something different, like talking sexy or going somewhere new for sex. She might be too bashful to discuss her desire, though, which is perhaps why the women's top wish list item was improved communication.
For some, establishing confidence is all that is necessary. People are highly accustomed to having their desires and fetishes mocked, chastised, and criticized. A guy must be honest about his own desires if he wants his girlfriend to share hers with him.

5. Role Play: According to 35% of women, having sex role-plays would strengthen marriages.
When two people pretend to be someone they're not, it's called role playing. They might even dress the role or act out a scene as two distinct characters. Some couples even go so far as to arrange their first meeting in public and center their entire story around a role play. It can be fun and empowering for couples who need to heat things up. Role play is different from acting out a sexual fantasy, because sometimes fantasies or fetishes don't require you to change your role.

Discuss a scenario you find interesting with her, and find out whether she has ever wished to be someone else or if she finds the thought of taking on a different role appealing. You can attempt acting out a situation you agree upon after talking about it. Here, consent is crucial! It's far preferable to plan ahead and question her beforehand in order to promote open communication.

No, Your Size Doesn't Matter

Size is completely unimportant to most women when it comes to their sexual enjoyment, according to numerous recent studies conducted over the years. It has nothing to do with size; rather, it has to do with how close you are to that person, how you get to know them, and other sensory details. People need to feel comfortable in their own skin, and that comfort can only come from within; size is completely irrelevant. What matters is the heart, the inner part.

No size is insignificant. The majority of women find enormous sizes to be extremely painful and uncomfortable, and it's all about enjoyment and pleasure. The ordinary woman also doesn't carry a tape measure in her hip pocket to measure penis sizes.
Once one understands a woman's physique, size becomes less significant and instead becomes technique, honesty, and desire.
It doesn't matter how big a guy is as long as he fulfills her requirements and isn't self-centered. This includes confidence in his own abilities as a person. What counts is how they proceed with other things to maximize a woman's enjoyment.

What counts is how they go about doing other things to maximize a woman's pleasure. As long as you provide their requirements in other areas, a woman will never view size as a priority.

It's pretty useless if you're huge and don't know how to use it.It works great regardless of size if you know how to use it, even if you're small.

While it is not everything, size does assist. Girth is more significant than length, but if you truly love the person you are with, everything else is secondary to the things they do and the way they make you feel on special occasions.
Because it is much more enjoyable in every sense, size does matter. However, wonderful intimacy is much more than just size.

Men have a skewed perception of what an average size is and believe that bigger is better, despite the fact that many women find that being huge is painful and uncomfortable. Women would just go right for the XL battery-powered devices and completely forgo dating if that was all that mattered.

Chapter Two: The Power of Quality Sex over Size

Particular Steps and Methods for Increasing Eroticism

Beyond the physical act of intimacy, some behaviors and methods create a shade of sensations. Through bringing these experiences into their interactions, couples open up new possibilities for increased fulfillment, exploratory discovery, and a deeper bond that goes beyond the norm. It's about turning the ordinary into the extraordinary and crafting a meaningful and unforgettable intimate story. The ability to perform these particular acts and procedures expertly, which enhance the shared experience between partners, is the art of intimacy as much as the physical acts.

1. Successful Interaction: One of the main components of increased sexual satisfaction is effective communication. Envision a situation where couples candidly talk about their fantasies, wants, and limits. Since both parties are in tune with each other's needs, wants, and boundaries, this conversation builds trust and paves the way for a more harmonious and satisfying experience.

2. Varied and Thoughtful Foreplay: When addressed creatively and thoughtfully, foreplay transcends the ordinary and becomes a vital component of the whole encounter. Imagine a scene where an engrossing massage, lighthearted taunting, or hushed remarks of expectation pave the way for an unforgettable and thrilling experience. These smart and varied foreplay techniques build suspense and foster an intimate setting.

3. A Knowledge of Erogenous Zones: Another factor contributing to increased happiness is the awareness of and concentration on particular erogenous zones. Imagine the delicate quality of a tender touch, the comforting afterglow of a kiss, or the thoughtful, individualized caresses. These little movements raise the level of arousal and intensify the pleasure that comes from the close relationship.

4. Developing Your Pacing and Rhythm: The intimate encounter gains dynamic quality from the skill of mastering rhythm and tempo. Imagine gliding between bursts of energy and calmer, more thoughtful movements with ease. This ebb and flow helps to maintain arousal throughout the session, keeping both parties interested and energized.

5. Trying Out Various Positions: By experimenting with different sexual positions, partners can customize their experiences to suit their own preferences. The variation provides energy to the interaction and encourages a sense of exploration and shared discovery, whether it is trying a new position for a deeper connection or finding solace in a time-honored favorite.

6. Conscientious Touch and Feeling: Beyond the physical act, the experience is elevated by mindful touch and heightened sensory awareness. Imagine a situation in which every contact is intentional and filled with awareness, concentrating on the physical characteristics of closeness. This level of intimacy raises the level of satisfaction that is gained from the shared experience as a whole.

7. Building a Bond Emotionally: The physical act becomes a meaningful connection when emotional closeness is infused into it. Imagine glances back and forth, hushed words of support, and sincere love creating an emotional environment that strengthens a couple's bond. The experience is elevated above the merely physical by this emotional resonance, resulting in a more meaningful and satisfying connection.

8. Examination of Shared Fantasy: A sense of shared adventure is created via the candid sharing and investigation of common fantasies. Imagine a situation in which couples feel free to explore and communicate their wishes, bringing a sense of adventure and excitement to the interaction. This reciprocal investigation leads to a more profound comprehension of one another's dreams, enhancing the general fulfillment that comes from the close relationship.

9. Ambience and Intuition: Adding unexpected features to personal interactions adds a spark of excitement and unpredictability. These unexpected elements, which can include venue changes, surprising gestures, or the addition of a new element to the routine, give the interaction an element of adventure and keep it lively and dynamic.

10. Ongoing Education and Adjustment: Envision a collaboration where participants are open to learning about one another's evolving requirements. The dynamic character of the close connection contributes to long-term enjoyment, as does the continuous process of learning and adjustment. A partnership in which parties are willing to learn about one other's changing desires.

Because of its flexibility, intimate experiences are certain to stay fresh and rewarding with every meeting.

The Benefits of Quality Sex and Its Power Over Size

There are several benefits to prioritizing quality sex over physical size in personal relationships that go well beyond appearances. Emotional connection, candid communication, and an emphasis on mutual satisfaction are characteristics of quality sex that cultivate an intimacy level that goes beyond physical characteristics.

The development and maintenance of an emotional bond between couples is at the center of this paradigm. The shared emotional experiences during intimate times are of great significance in quality sex, in contrast to the belief that size determines satisfaction.

A stronger, more durable relationship foundation is bolstered by the relationships created via emotional connection. In addition to the physical act, partners who have high-quality sexual experiences also feel great fulfillment in the shared vulnerability and trust that these relationships foster.

Effective communication about preferences, boundaries, and desires is essential to having enjoyable sex. Good sex partners regularly participate in talks that go beyond social norms, fostering an environment that is comfortable for candid discussion.

This dialogue opens the door to a more profound and pleasurable experience for both parties by facilitating a deeper knowledge of one another. Quality sex puts an emphasis on communication, which helps partners align their expectations and creates a respectful and trusting environment.

The emphasis on reciprocal exploration in great sex is one of its unique features. Couples are encouraged to investigate each other's bodies and wants rather than focusing on preconceived notions or expectations. This investigation develops a feeling of adventure and freshness in the connection in addition to adding an exciting element. Variety and flexibility are essential to quality sex, as is accepting the possibility of ongoing exploration and realizing that preferences may change over time.

The ongoing satisfaction that comes from having good sex is noteworthy when it comes to long-term relationships. Intimacy can be sustained over time with quality sex, unlike the transient appeal of physical qualities. In order to ensure that partners continue to feel fulfillment, it acts as a dynamic force that changes with the partnership to make sure that partners keep finding fulfillment in their experiences together. Good sex adds to the overall happiness and durability of a relationship by fostering an enduring bond between partners.

Furthermore, healthy physical characteristic comparisons and competition are discouraged by excellent sex. Without needless pressure or condemnation, couples can value one other's distinctive characteristics by reorienting the focus to emotional connection and shared satisfaction. This method creates a pleasant sexual atmosphere that helps people feel more confident and have a positive body image.

Another important benefit of putting excellent sex first is the decrease in performance anxiety. When partners enjoy satisfying sexual encounters, they are freed from the pressure to live up to societal norms regarding physical appearance. This freedom makes it possible to communicate desire and pleasure more honestly, which promotes a more carefree and joyful intimate relationship.

To put it briefly, good sex becomes a significant factor in close relationships. With benefits that go far beyond the apparent limitations of physical size, it honors the beauty of emotional connection, clear communication, and mutual discovery. It is an investment in continuing closeness that creates a long-lasting, exciting, and satisfying sexual connection.

Beholders have different perceptions of size. Many factors, such as cultural standards, the kind of sex one is experiencing, one's own sexual demands, and many others, influence people's preferences for genital size.
Studies indicate that most people's sexual preferences are not primarily influenced by size. 84% of women said they were happy with their partner's penis size in a study of 52,031 heterosexual men and women some years back. The percentage of people who desired their partner's penis to be bigger or smaller was only 14% and 2%, respectively.

Sometimes, the size of the penis might influence certain things, such as:

Sexual comfort: Penetration may be uncomfortable if the penis is too big for the partner, especially if there isn't enough lubricant. It may be very difficult or perhaps impossible to have anal intercourse if there are large size differences.

Sexual pleasure: A person's capacity to arouse their partner may be influenced by the length and circumference of their penis. A person with a small but wide penis, for instance, might be able to stimulate a partner's anus or vagina significantly, but they might not be able to reach deeper locations.

Perceptions and sexual anxiety: Size is not the only thing that matters. The impression of the ideal size of a penis held by each partner may have an impact on how much fun they have. For instance, even if one's penis is average in size, one may experience anxiety due to the perception of a small penis.

Quality Sex Has Benefits Over Penis Size

Prioritizing quality sex over body size emerges as a transformational paradigm that creates genuine connection and transcends societal standards in a world where physical beauty is typically the focus. Let's dissect this idea and examine the many benefits that result from emphasizing the depth of the sexual experience as opposed to flimsy details like physical attributes.

The understanding that good sex places a significant emphasis on the emotional bond between lovers is at the core of the benefits. A good sexual relationship is built on emotional connection rather than the transient appeal of physical size. When partners have quality sex, they travel a path of trust and vulnerability, creating relationships that go beyond the physical act and into the domain of mutual understanding and emotions.

One of the mainstays of the quality sex paradigm is effective communication. It involves more than just voicing wants; it also entails establishing a forum for candid communication. Good sex teaches partners how to respectfully and sensitively handle discussions about fantasies, boundaries, and desires. This degree of communication encourages vulnerability and trust, two qualities that are necessary for a more satisfying intimate connection.

In the world of good sex, getting to know each other's bodies and wants becomes a joyful adventure. Couples are urged to accept and celebrate each other's individual preferences rather than giving in to social pressures related to physical appearance. This investigation adds excitement and freshness to the partnership, going beyond mere physical fulfillment adding an element of excitement and novelty to the relationship as partners discover new facets of intimacy.

A notable sustaining factor in long-term relationships is high-quality sex. Quality sex becomes an enduring investment in the connection experienced by lovers, unlike the fleeting appeal of body size. It functions as a dynamic element of the partnership, developing and adjusting throughout time to the shifting circumstances. The benefits also include preserving contentment and closeness while spouses move through different phases of their joint adventure.

Most importantly, putting excellent sex first frees people from the needless stress of body-size comparison and rivalry. The focus moves from following social norms to finding happiness in shared activities. This change in emphasis promotes a healthy sexual environment, which helps both partners feel more confident and have a favorable body image.

Another significant benefit of having wonderful sex is that it lessens performance anxiety. When partners enjoy satisfying sexual encounters, they are freed from the burden of meeting societal standards related to physical appearance. This release makes it easier to express desire and pleasure more authentically, which promotes relaxation and enjoyment during close relationships.

The benefits of choosing quality over quantity of sex are essentially transformational. This paradigm offers advantages that go much beyond the expectations of society regarding physical attractiveness. It celebrates the beauty of emotional connection, efficient communication, and mutual exploration.
It encourages people to delve into the many facets of intimacy and develop a relationship that values depth and genuineness. Partners who adopt this paradigm discover a new depth of contentment and fulfillment in their close relationships, which is based on the transforming potential of high-quality sex.

Chapter Three: Techniques for Sensational Sex Regardless of Your Size

All guys feel amazing when they make a girl lose control in bed for some reason! However, it's not unexpected that many men desire to know the finest sex advice for men that can quickly stimulate and satisfy women, as no one truly teaches men these things.
It takes more than simply penetration to make love to a woman. Warming up takes time for women. Furthermore, you cannot rush the procedure unless she has already been aroused.

You may feel like a rock star in bed with these tongue twisters, pelvic thrusts, and sex positions. Unfortunately, because every woman is different, not every one of these motions works perfectly. Furthermore, a woman's attraction to one person may repel another.

Perhaps you want to improve your ability to satisfy your lover, perhaps you want to heighten the intensity of your orgasms, lengthen your erections, and spend more time in bed. Perhaps you'd want to learn more about anal play, whether sex toys are ideal for couples, or how to discuss your darkest, most intense sexual dreams with your partner.

Maybe you're bored with your current relationship and want to try your hand at BDSM (Bondage and Discipline, Domination and Submission, Sadism and Masochism) or perhaps thinking about dating someone else. Whatever the issue, there's a good chance you'll find advice that will be helpful. Because they address more than just particulars, the sex advice that follows won't ever land you in hot water in the bedroom due to your size.

In case you're in a committed relationship with a lady, you might already be aware of what makes her feel attracted to you in bed and what doesn't. You can leverage this knowledge, together with these suggestions, to your benefit.
Instead of concentrating on positions or hard sex, though, if you're just hitting it off with a female for the first time, follow these suggestions for sex and you'll have her groaning and gripping the sheets in no time!

Tips to Increase Your Sexual Pleasure

Men who think that their penises are too little can benefit from a number of techniques. Some advice and ideas are as follows:

1. Recognizing that their partners may not be concerned about their penis size

2. Being aware that anxiety about penis thickness does not always indicate that a person has a thin penis

3. Concentrating on alternative methods of pleasing a spouse, such stimulating the penis or clitoral area giving oral sex priority

4. Considering anal sex

5. Trying out sex toys during pre- and post-sex

6. Practicing candid communication with partners

7. Expressing worries to a spouse regarding penis size so they can provide reassurances

8. Playing around with new sexual positions, such approaching a lover from behind

9. Trying various approaches to entering a partner with furniture, cushions, or other things

10. To give the impression that the penis is thicker, try entering a partner from the side or back or in other postures that keep their legs together.

Techniques for Sensational Sex to Make Her Happy.

1. Remain clean and fresh.
Take care of yourself down there. As long as you keep your beard tidy, you don't have to entirely shave.
Take a shower before going to bed if you're having sex after a strenuous and sweaty workday. If you want to initiate some foreplay before bed, you can encourage her to take a quick shower. Little things have the power to have a great impact.

2. Foreplay:
One of the most significant sex advice pieces for men is this. Don't rush into her right away. Recall that girls need some time to become fully aroused and prepared for sexual activity.
Even if she's just ready for penetration, she might not like it as much if you take your time indulging

in foreplay. Penetrating her when she's dry or barely aroused could injure her.

3. Take notice of her erogenous zones.
The sensitive areas of a woman's body are known as her erogenous zones. Licking or nibbling her erogenous zones can quickly make her feel hot and uncomfortable, even if she's not feeling particularly confident or in the mood.
You may tell how eager she will be for sex in a matter of minutes by placing your lips on her earlobes, neck, nape, elbows, forearms, underarms, or pelvis.

4 Don't rush into sexual activity.
Sexuality isn't like a race. Before engaging in sexual activity, spend some time getting to know your companion. You and your spouse can learn what works and what doesn't in bed together, in addition to increasing desire."Sex is a somewhat mechanical activity on its own.

Keep from getting too close to her. Don't start tossing her back and forth just yet; instead, gently touch her down there with your member and mock her by sneaking it in sometimes. Before you go all the way into her, make her want it extremely badly.

A girl will beg you for it in desperation if you tease her in bed, and you'll quickly drive her insane.

5. Explore her body:
Her mound and her boobs might have your full attention. However, there is a tonne more you can do to pique her interest. When you first get into bed, avoid putting your hands directly in her vulnerable spots.
You can approach her breasts after you've tasted and lingered on every part of her body by letting your hands and lips roam over her entire body. She would go insane with the wait and the excitement!

6. Inhale deeply into her
When you're making love to her, bring your face up to hers. And press your face against her neck while taking a big inhale through your nose.
As long as she thinks him appealing, women are quickly aroused by a man's scent and pheromones. During sex, breathing deeply close to her earlobes fosters more intimacy and intensifies sexual desire.

7. Close your eyes or make eye contact.
When you're above her, look into her eyes. She'll develop a stronger sense of connection and love for you. However, simply close your eyes and relish the enjoyable feeling if the glances get uncomfortable.

She'll worry whether you're bored already, so try not to wander about the room or stare at anything else but the female.

8. Follow her lead
When you're having sex with her, try to read her thoughts. It's best to avoid asking too many questions during a sexual encounter because unclear answers and questions themselves can be major distractions and sap the enthusiasm from the moment.
She enjoys what you're doing if her groans get more intense. She wants you to move quicker if she shifts her pelvis more quickly.
Try to establish an emotional connection with her throughout your intercourse, and just go with the flow. She will feel closer to you since she will believe that you are aware of her needs.

9. Get down on her.
One of the most crucial pieces of advice for men having sex is to never be egocentric in bed. You can bet that a female who enjoys getting laid will also like having sex with you.
When engaging in oral foreplay, don't make it appear like it's always a lead-up to sex; instead, use it as a prelude.

In between sex, you may occasionally even pull out of her and lay down on her for a short while. Your tongue would be a great substitute for your member for a short while, since she's already wet.

10. Acquire the skill of delaying sex
How much time can you spend in bed? You're probably not at your fittest right now if you can't hold your own for at least 20 minutes on a typical day.

11. Continue to exert yourself more for longer
Exercise to increase your stamina. Exercise offers you a fantastic body and increases blood circulation, which leads to firmer erections and more stamina.
When you take off your clothes, you'll feel more self-assured, she'll adore you more for your extreme good looks, and you'll remain fierce for a lot longer. Any way you slice it, that's good news.

You're not the only one who wishes to prolong sex. Almost all men experience premature ejaculation at some point in their lives.
You can postpone ejaculation by using kegel exercises. Encouraging your pelvic floor's pubococcygeal (PC) muscles will help you better regulate your sex-induced orgasms.

12. Don't worry about the tiny man
Avoid obsessing over your erection, since this could
cause it to vanish before you ever get close to her.
Simply concentrate on enjoying your partner *or
your hookup*, and your little guy will rise to the
occasion when he needs to perform.

It's vital to remember that if you're having trouble
getting the little man to stand, especially after
extended foreplay sessions, it could be a mental
trick.
Just relax; he'll be prepared for the duty when it
comes.

13. Use dirty language and give in to fantasies
Don't allow the back and forth action in bed with
your spouse to get too monotonous. Talk to her
from time to time, telling her how lovely she looks
and feels on your body.
And to push the boundaries even farther, talk to her
about a sexual desire you have. If she finds what
you say interesting, she will definitely start
urinating on the bed shortly! Are you curious about
whether your significant other enjoys having shady
conversations? Use a phrase like "You make me
think dirty thoughts." Take it gradually at first.
Instead of diving straight in with your dirtiest, most

intimate conversation right away, it's better to tread
lightly.

14. Mix it up
Every now and then, accelerate, and then return to
the deliberate, sluggish grind. She will become even
more aroused if you vary your movements in bed
and give her an unexpected, abrupt change in
speed.
There is nothing worse than having boring sex,
therefore never let it happen.
Occasionally pick up the pace or shift the topic of
conversation. She will adore you more the more
creative you are in bed.

15. Make use of your hands
In bed, avoid leaving your hands unoccupied. Even
after you've penetrated her, move your hands over
her body. Don't just put your hand behind her back
and hold it there the entire time as support.
You can grip her butt or slip your hands over her
back and move them over her breasts. She will love
it when you use your hands a lot during sex.

16. Give it a go.
Try something different with your partner if you've
been having sex in a certain style for some time to
see if you both enjoy it. Even while your silent

missionary job seems ideal right now, if you don't
do something different every once in a while, it will
become monotonous quickly.
Play dress-up, speak dirty, have sultry sex, or
indulge in a few steamy kinky fantasies in bed.

17. Find out what interests her.
Inquiring about her preferences in bed is a smart
idea whether or not you're in a new relationship.
While some women enjoy having their breasts
caressed, others do not. Some people can only
orgasm when they're on top, while others never
orgasm at all.

She will be quite appreciative if you ask her what
feels nice and what she wants done to her. The
majority of males never even ask.
Rather, they are self-centered and merely consider
what will make them happy. Thus, demonstrating
your desire to please her will make you stand out
from the crowd, which is why this is also the best
sex advice for men.

18. Establish the tone
It is not necessary to stop there—we just discussed
how music can create a romantic atmosphere for
sex. To create a cozier atmosphere, burn candles,
prepare a bubble bath, or acquire silk linens. You

see, women enjoy a romantic atmosphere. They truly want a caring and affectionate environment when they are having sex with a man since women are more emotional than men are. It demonstrates that he values her highly enough to make an attempt to enhance the romance of their sexual encounter.

19. Give sex toys a try
Now, unless you two really want to, you don't have to get too crazy with these! You might start out easy, say by using a vibrator to play. She may even have one already, and you will likely win her over if you offer to use it during sex because many women find it impossible to orgasm without one.
Other than vibrators, there are plenty of other choices. To find out what you both want to try, you may even go to an X-rated store or shop online.

From modest to truly extravagant, there are countless alternatives. In any case, if your routine has become too monotonous, it adds something fresh.

20. Take up role-playing.
Although roleplaying demands a great deal of suspension of disbelief, the rewards can be enormous if you can give it your all. Numerous

well-known roles—such as boss/secretary,
teacher/student, and stripper/customer—play on
the idea that one is in charge and the other is at
their mercy.
Even in happy and healthy sexual relationships,
these are powerful dynamics. They give the [lovers]
the freedom to act out their dreams without making
them feel exposed.

When two individuals have been together for a long
time, role playing might be beneficial. There are
times when all you want is to "be with someone
else." Consequently, you can spend time with your
companion as you both perform.
Anything from a teacher/student drama to a
cop/prison drama could be the subject.
Alternatively, you may go to a bar and take seats at
opposing ends.
Act as though you don't know one another, and
when you "pretend" to meet, improvise. Play the
part of two strangers who meet, go home, and
engage in passionate sex with your "new" partner.

21. Occasionally quickies
Yes, ladies enjoy long, passionate sex that is
accompanied by music and candles. Real life,
meanwhile, sometimes leaves you with little time
for all of that. Many people are unable to spend

hours on end having sex because of their jobs, children, or any other ordinary obligations.
Thus, don't be scared to indulge in quickies! They are also liked by women. Quickies can actually be extremely fervent and animalistic. You have the overwhelming need to have the person in this now, right now.

22. Use your tongue wisely
Avoid using your tongue like a dart during a kiss (in and out, in and out). Instead, experiment with different pressure levels and movements.

23. Give a cock ring a try.
 The cock ring is the "superfood of sex toys" due to its affordability, simplicity of usage, and wide range of benefits for your sexual life. You may improve your erection, increase your self-confidence, and intensify your orgasms with a tight ring that fits around the base of your penis (and occasionally your testicles, too). Choosing a vibrating alternative may also aid in clitoris or booty stimulation for your companion.

24. Engage in mutual masturbation.
Too frequently, we define "sex" as having the penis in the vagina or the anus, but that's such a narrow definition of what sex is. Now engage in mutual

masturbation, which involves masturbating with your partner. You get to see how your spouse touches themself, which is a bonus. It's also fantastic for when you're too exhausted to get it on. That way, you can touch them precisely how they want the next time you have partnered sex!

25. Look for a condom that fits well.
You may not be using the correct condoms if you detest how they make you feel during intercourse. As per the sex therapist Choose a condom that fits like a glove and keep an eye out for ribbed rubbers. It's important to pick the condom that feels the greatest for you because they are quite effective at avoiding STIs and pregnancy.

26. Explore temperature play. The method known as "temperature play" involves applying heat or cold to the skin to elicit a sexual response.
In order to create a strong sensory response, you can either rub an ice cube over your partner's body (the boudoir is particularly sensitive to heat) or engage in wax play.

27. Use anal beads or a butt plug.
In addition to stimulating the prostate during partner intercourse or masturbation, these butt-centric sex toys can also prick the sensitive

nerve endings at the anus hole. Anal beads can be progressively inserted or removed throughout a sex session, whereas butt plugs are made to slip in and stay in place—thus the name plu

28. Lubricate up.
Lubrication increases the comfort and speed with which you can penetrate the vagina and grind against the clitoris, but sometimes, no matter how turned on a woman might be psychologically, she can have trouble getting wet. This is the role of lubricant. Before engaging in sexual activity, try squeezing a few drops onto the tip of your penis.

29. Watch obscene content together.
Let us share with you a little secret: many women enjoy watching porn. In a Men's Health survey, 75% of women stated that they would not mind watching porn while having sex or during foreplay. However, keep in mind that they might not enjoy the same stuff as you do, so be sure to explore some softer-core options or talk about your preferences in advance.

30. During foreplay, don't instantly turn south.
The genitalia are not to be touched during foreplay. Utilizing your fingers, a feather, a silk scarf, or anything else that piques their interest, touch the

various areas of their body and inquire as to how it feels. This keeps the tension building until you both feel like exploding.

31. Circle the clitoris of your spouse.
When it comes to climaxing, P-in-V intercourse is probably insufficient for a vulva partner; they will likely want clitoral stimulation. So how can you get your partner's clitoris to become more active? When a partner draws circles on their clitoris with their fingers or tongue, three out of four women who participated in an Indiana University poll of 1,055 said they liked it. Conversely, ask your partner what makes them tick if you're not quite sure!

32. Nevertheless, avoid making too much clitoral touch.
Your lover might object if you make direct contact with them in the clitoris because it's extremely sensitive and nerve-racking. It's possible to massage the clitoris without exerting direct pressure because it really extends several inches beneath the skin on either side of the vagina, much like a wishbone. Use lubricant and try tracing the extensions with gentle, zigzagging finger movements or flat, wide, extra-wet tongue strokes.

Next, slowly work your way around the top in a spiral, getting closer each time.
Those pleasure centers will come to life through the anticipation and indirect interaction combined.

33. Close the pleasure gap as well as the orgasm gap.
It's admirable that you want to facilitate your partner's climax because the orgasm gap is real! However, if you make it the only thing on your mind during a sexual encounter—for example, by telling them you won't come until they're ready—you risk making them anxious and reducing the chance that they will experience an orgasm.

34. Never ask your partner if they finished
"Did you come?" is a question you should never ask someone who has a vulva after sex. You're subtly telling your spouse that their enjoyment is an afterthought for you if you ask that question after sex instead of during the act, and that's not acceptable. Rather, during the actual sex, prioritize their pleasure.

35. Change locations
Many people develop a pattern of exclusively having sex in their beds. It may be cozy, but the experience isn't necessarily thrilling. Thus, vary your places.

Try the floor in the bathroom, the shower, the kitchen table, and the couch.

Another option is to attempt it in a "forbidden" location away from your residences. You could join the mile high club, do it in an abandoned movie theater, or in a field beneath the stars. Just take care not to get discovered or arrested!

36. Every lady is unique

This is a crucial matter. Not every girl has the same tastes in bed; each one is different. Not every female will respond the same way to music or dirty chatting, even if it has worked well for you. As you engage in sexual activity with her, observe her reactions to your actions and attempt to ascertain her preferences by observing her movements in bed. It's the simplest method for determining what matters and what doesn't.

Tailoring Techniques for Varied Preferences and Experience Levels

1. Recognizing Diverse Preferences: Partners should be honest with each other about their individual dreams, boundaries, and desires. This conversation guarantees that the personal experience is tailored

to suit each person's tastes. Recognize that everyone's preferences, aversions, and degree of comfort in private settings vary.

2. Personalization of Foreplay Methods: While some people might love a sultry massage, others might prefer lighthearted conversation or vocal declarations of desire. Partners can create a setting that meets a range of sensory and emotional needs by personalizing foreplay.The prelude to intimacy is called foreplay, and it should be customized to each partner's tastes in both comfort and excitement.

3. Changing the Rhythm and Pace: People with differing degrees of experience could feel more or less at ease. By changing the cadence, you may make the experience more comfortable for those who are new to intimacy and interesting for those who are seasoned. Intimate experiences should be paced according to how both people feel.

4. Diverse Position Exploration: Partners may have varying degrees of comfort and experience in various roles. Diverse tastes are accommodated by examining a range of stances, some of which emphasize emotional connection and others of which offer diversity and surprise.Various positions provide varying degrees of comfort and contentment.

5. Sensation Tailored to Preferences: Sensation tailored to preferences takes into account personal preferences; some people may prefer gentle caresses, while others may be drawn to more powerful experiences. The variety of desires in the intimate relationship is respected and welcomed by this customized approach. Touch ought to be considerate and customized to each person's preferences.

6. Establishing a Deeper Emotional Bond via a Range of Expressions: A deeper emotional bond can

be achieved through a range of expressions, including vocal affirmations, compassionate gestures, and shared laughing. It is important for partners to find expressions that suit their individual comfort zones. Communicate feelings in a way that both partners find comfortable.

7. Promoting the Exploration of Diverse Fantasies: It's critical to establish a secure environment for talking about and investigating a variety of fantasies. Respecting each partner's individual aspirations, whether it's through a first-time exploration or the realization of long-held desires, an inclusive approach is important. It's acceptable to have diverse desires, and couples ought to feel comfortable examining them together.

8. Surprise and Spontaneity Adapted to Comfort Levels: Although some people might find surprise actions entertaining, others might need a more routine setting. Customizing surprises guarantees

that they are both thrilling and considerate of personal preferences. Surprises should be thrilling but also stay within each partner's comfort zones.

9. Constant Learning and Adaptation as an Inclusive mentality: An inclusive mentality calls for constant dialogue around changing limits and desires. In order to guarantee a constantly fulfilling and inclusive experience, partners must modify their methods. Continue getting to know one another's preferences and be flexible.

Recognizing and appreciating the unique qualities that every partner offers to the relationship is part of a customized approach to intimacy. Partners may create a space where intimacy is not only pleasurable but also inclusive and respectful of each other's distinct journeys and comfort levels by customizing experiences to suit individual tastes and accommodating shifting desires.

Chapter Four: Breaking Taboos: Uncensored Sex Secrets That is Not About Size

Uncensored Sexual Secrets: Adding Momentum to the Sexual Pleasure

Unrestricted sexual secrets can lead to a more happy and thrilling personal relationship. Partners can discover new levels of excitement and depth in their sexual journey by breaking taboos, exploring fantasies, understanding individual preferences, incorporating sensory exploration, embracing spontaneity, mastering teasing, prioritizing mutual pleasure, and engaging in continuous exploration. An intimate connection becomes more lively and thrilling when partners are willing to explore the raw parts of desire. This is because it provides freshness and enhances the tie between them.

Breaking Taboos and Starting a Conversation: Uncensored sex secrets frequently entail breaking taboos and starting a conversation about fantasies and desires. Breaking down social conventions and creating a welcoming atmosphere allows partners to talk openly about their most private, often strange, wants. This openness creates the groundwork for a more sincere and thrilling close relationship.

Investigating Fantasy Realms: Adding excitement to the sexual experience can be achieved with the help of fantasy. Spoken sex secrets allow lovers to freely discuss and experience their craziest dreams without fear of repercussions. Experimenting with power dynamics, role-playing, or traveling to exciting places—being able to freely explore these raw desires adds a fresh and exciting element to a close relationship.

Understanding Individual Preferences: The significance of comprehending and honoring individual preferences is underscored in Uncensored Sex Secrets. Open communication about what genuinely thrills and fulfills a partner is encouraged. This degree of comprehension enables a customized approach to intimacy, where each partner's wishes are respected, resulting in a more exciting and unique encounter.

Including Sensory Exploration: A greater emphasis on sensory exploration is frequently seen in uncensored sex secrets. Partners can enter a world of enhanced sensations by embracing sensory-enhancing objects like blindfolds or shackles, experimenting with various textures and temperatures, and more. The personal voyage is made much more exciting and pleasurable by this sensory adventure.

Accepting variation and Spontaneity: Uncensored Sex Secrets embrace variation and spontaneity. It's suggested for couples to embrace the unexpected and break out from habit. The element of surprise and diversity infuses a feeling of adventure into the personal relationship, guaranteeing that each meeting seems new and thrilling, whether it's by introducing surprises, attempting new positions, or exploring various settings.

Learning the Art of Teasing: Teasing is a potent component of uninhibited sex secrets when it is done without hesitation. Playful repartee, extended waiting, or enticing touches can all be used by partners to create suspense. The build-up to intimate moments is made more exciting and dynamic by this art of teasing, which heightens the whole experience.

Prioritizing Mutual Pleasure: The significance of putting mutual pleasure first is shown by uncensored sex secrets. It is recommended that couples concentrate on making each other happy while experimenting with methods and behaviors that increase pleasure. A reciprocal dynamic is created by this shared engagement in pleasure, which deepens the connection and amplifies the excitement of the intimate interactions overall.

Engaging in continuous exploration: Uncensored sex secrets are a journey that we are always exploring. It is encouraged for partners to constantly investigate and uncover new facets of their boundaries and wants. This ongoing exploration makes sure that the sexual adventure is dynamic, changing to suit changing tastes and keeping things exciting for the duration of the relationship.

Uncensored Sexual Secrets

1. Intense Nipple Play

The primary purpose of the breast, an external organ, is to nourish (lactate) a woman's kids. However, the breast performs other "functions" besides breastfeeding, as you are probably well aware of. Specifically, you can arouse your spouse during erotic play by using the breast.

However, the areola and the nipple are more sensitive to touch than the actual breast.

The pigmented skin around the nipples is called the areola. Because the areola is so touch-sensitive, you can use it to great use in your nipple play adventures.

The nipple, the jewel in the breast's crown, is located in the center of the areola.

There are countless techniques to make your lover or yourself feel good about your nipples, including caressing, nibbling, fondling, and vibrating.

A fun foreplay session should include some good breast play. But for the most part, heavy nipple play is still frowned upon.

Nipple stimulation alone has the power to induce an orgasm in the majority of women.You must exercise patience, focus, and even creativity.

An orgasm that starts at the nipple is known as a nipple orgasm. A clitoral orgasm and this one are comparable in intensity since most of the throbs happen at the nipple. An especially sensitive erogenous zone is the nipples. Arousal has been associated with regions of the body known as erogenous zones.

In total, there are seven of them; they are as follows:

Lips

Ears

Neck

Buttocks and lower back

Breasts and nipples

Inside the thighs

Clitoris

These locations can provide your companion unbelievably intense pleasure when stimulated just properly.

It is highly recommended that you spend some time in your partner's other erogenous zones. However, if you want to rapidly send your woman to her knees, you should concentrate on the nipples because they are extremely sensitive.

Nipple Play: Advanced Tips and Techniques

Nipple clamps

Nipple clamps are another "must try" sex device if your partner is a little more daring.

The main function of a sex toy called a "nipple clamp" is to increase sensitivity by trapping blood within the tissues.

Nipple clamps are fantastic since they provide a hands-free method of satisfying your partner's desires, allowing you to concentrate on other things.

As you transition from sucking to other activities, use nipple clamps to maintain your partner's nipples' sensitivity. Alternately, combine them with sucking for a more powerful effect.

Nipple Pumps

A small device that is positioned around the nipple is called a nipple pump. The pump mechanism, which can be electric or manual, is either attached to a tube or located at the tip of the pump.

A vacuum is produced when the pump is turned on. The nipples will feel the attraction of this vacuum, which will raise pressure. Blood flow to the nipples will consequently rise. Both engorgement and heightened sensitivity result from this.

Then you can give her a great deal of pleasure by using the preceding sucking and playing advice.

Titty Fuck

Whatever you name it, mammary intercourse, breast sex, boob bang, or titty wank, it's really awesome.

Here's are some titty fuck tips to completely satisfy your spouse sexually.

1. Chest Straddle (Cock to Mouth) is one of the best titty wank positions.

2. Ass to Mouth Reverse Chest Straddle

3. Bending over Tit Wank

4. Tit Wank Lying

5. Tit Wank Sideways

6. Modified 69

2. Masturbating in Front of Your Partner

Many people learn early on that masturbating is improper, embarrassing, and should be done in private. One of the greatest anxieties that most people retain from youth into adulthood is being discovered to be masturbating. And even in very loving, committed relationships, most people find it too awkward to masturbate in front of their partner.

But there are lots of benefits to breaking this. Engaging in a behavior you often keep private in front of your significant other can foster intimacy and trust. Masturbating tends to make you feel embarrassed and ashamed, but you quickly get over it and your relationship gets stronger. Getting what you want in bed can also be accomplished more quickly and effectively by masturbating in front of your partner. You can demonstrate to your partner the kinds of movement and touch that you find enjoyable. It will undoubtedly improve your foreplay and sex tremendously and can even turn into mutual masturbation if you so desire.

3. Having Sex With Toys

It's entertaining to breach the typical "forbidden act" of using sex toys during sexual activity. Many people think it would be impolite to use a toy during intercourse with your spouse, as if you were telling them you weren't happy. However, some of the best sex ever can result from it.

Common positions such as missionary, cowgirl, and doggy may become otherworldly experiences with a basic clit or wand vibrator, resulting in full body, shaking orgasms.

4. Outdoor Sexual

One of the most thrilling taboo sex acts you may violate is alfresco sex. Exciting outdoor sex is guaranteed, whether you prefer quickies or oral sex. Please note that it may be against the law in your area to have sex in a public setting or anywhere accessible to the general public. Because of this, a remote beach is the ideal location for outdoor sexual activity—as long as no one can observe!

5. Exhibitionism

A large portion of the excitement surrounding outdoor sex stems from "exhibitionism," the phenomenon in which one becomes aroused by being observed by others in the nude or engaging in sexual activity. There are various ways to legally and safely expose yourself to people without their consent, even if it's against the law and considered a sexual offense.

Consider having a "Peeping Tom" (as seen above) or someone you can trust to keep an eye on you when you and your spouse are having intimate moments. You might enjoy trying cam sex if you're feeling particularly daring and you and your partner are game. You could get a kick out of having people watch you get personal.

6. Voyeurism

It is strictly forbidden to see someone else without their consent or to take pictures or videos of them without their consent. Non-consensual voyeurism is a type of sexual abuse. Nevertheless, as long as the subject gives permission, it's acceptable to become aroused when you witness someone else—like your partner—in the nude or participating in sexual activity.

There are several methods to incorporate voyeurism into your sexual encounters. Observing your spouse during a masturbation is a terrific method to find out more about the kinds of touch and sensations they find enjoyable. You might enjoy seeing them engage in sexual activity with another person, such as a friend, partner, or even a sex worker.

7. Massage of the Anals

Booty play is undoubtedly more acceptable now than it was in the past, but most people still view "venturing south" as forbidden. Anal massage is among the more gentle measures. For all genders, it's an excellent foreplay act that delivers increased pleasure and larger orgasms.

It could be helpful to start viewing the butt as an erogenous surface, similar to a nipple, rather than as a hole if you or your spouse are a little uncomfortable with butt materials. By deciding to spend all of your time outside, you can both unwind and enjoy yourselves without feeling pressured. You are about to enter a whole new world of pleasure.

Start by gently massaging the butt and perineum with a finger or toy that has been well-lubricated.

8. Rimming

Giving and receiving an anal massage feels great, but nothing compares to the satisfaction of eating your ass or "rimming" Using your tongue to lick your partner's butthole is a delightful foreplay act that feels great, regardless of your sexual orientation, even though it's still frowned upon by most people.

Showering or using an antiseptic wipe is a must for the receiving partner before rimming. To provide endless pleasure, the "giver" can coat their partner's asshole with tasty lubricant and begin licking, caressing, and playing with it.

9. BDSM and bondage

Bondage sex can be far more stimulating than intimate, romantic sex, even though it still feels amazing. Bondage sex is worth indulging in if you've always dreamed about tying your spouse up or being bound yourself.

BDSM, which stands for bondage, discipline, dominance, and submission, includes bondage sex. Generally, it entails blindfolding, teasing, and carefully restraint your partner. You may also incorporate powerful stimulation techniques like stroking, tickling, and oral sex. Impact play is not always the result of bondage sex, although it can be.

Any object you have on hand, such as a belt, silk scarf, or necktie, can be used for impromptu bondage sex, but you should always establish a safe word beforehand. Tie bows rather than knots as a precaution since the former can be quickly undone. Additionally, always maintain a one-finger space between your partner's skin and the restriction.

10. Impact Act

The thought of slapping, spanking, or even whipping your lover can be alluring once you've tied them up. This is one of the most thrilling taboos you can break; it's called impact play. Before experimenting with any kind of impact play, you should establish and follow a safe word, just like with bondage and BDSM sex. This will maintain the atmosphere of pleasure and consent.

Impact play doesn't require you to tie your partner up, although it certainly helps. I advise taking things one step at a time, beginning with some light spanking.

11. Being Degraded

Being degraded can be your ideal sex act if you find pleasure and humiliation to be attractive. Since rough sex allows you to safely explore your thoughts and internalized shame, it's one of the best ways to feel "used."

If you've always secretly longed to be treated like a piece of useless garbage.

12. Choking

Choking is one of the most effective BDSM play techniques, but it can also be one of the riskiest if you don't know what you're doing. While it gives you a heated, strong sense of being subjugated and dominated, choking fosters connection and trust. A wonderful surge can be experienced when someone you trust briefly restricts your airway.

It should never be necessary to obstruct or restrict your partner's airways; instead, choking must be consensual. It is preferable to place your hand on your partner's upper chest as opposed to their neck or throat. It's better to give your partner the impression of being choked rather than the actual chokehold.

13. Spitting

If you want to be domineering, spitting in your partner's mouth or on their body can be a great turn-on. If it's with a person you trust sexually, being on the receiving end can be a sweet way to demonstrate surrender and foster trust. On the other hand, it can also appear demeaning.

14. Trios

Having a threesome was one of the most popularly desired taboo sex practices, in my experience. Threesomes are the ultimate taboo for many, whether you're single and want to join a couple or in a relationship and want to bring a buddy.

15. Swinging

Although most people consider it inappropriate, having sex with someone you are not in a relationship with is quite common. If both partners are receptive to the concept, learning about the swingers' way of life might revitalize a committed partnership.

One safe method for couples to "hard swap" is through sex clubs and parties. It's crucial to continue talking both before and after the sex and to always have safe sexual behavior.

16. Spouting

Squirting is one of the most embarrassing and taboo female bodily processes, even though it's normal and natural. Very little research has been done on this phenomena. Most women squirt when their G-spot is touched, but some can also squirt when their clitoris is rubbed, and some can squirt when their anals are aroused.

17. Anal Intercourse

Even for individuals who are receptive to anal massage or rimming, anal sex is still considered a "off-limits" behavior, even though it's no longer as taboo as it once was. Many people associate "anal sex" with deep, thrusting, "porn-like" penetration when they hear the term. However, mild penetration of the anal region can be an excellent "ingredient" in the bedroom, increasing the intensity and ease of orgasms.

There are several little-known advantages of anal sex for both men and women. It causes men's P-spot, or prostate, to become stimulated, which can result in pleasurable P-spot orgasms. When paired with clitoral and G-spot stimulation (with a finger or toy), anal intercourse for women can cause intense orgasms and even squirting since it stimulates their A-spot, which is located near their cervix.

18. Pegging

Pegging, which is quickly gaining popularity, is what anal sex was twenty years ago. It describes the act of a woman penetrating her male companion anally with a strap-on dildo. It's a beautiful, personal gesture that can make any wife or girlfriend feel more connected to her husband or partner. It can strengthen any couple's bond and calls for a great deal of trust.

Pegging can cause strong P-spot orgasms in males, exactly like anal intercourse, and it's equally thrilling for women.

Women who have tried it report extremely hot and powerful sensations of sensuality. They can experience incredible clitoral and G-spot stimulation simultaneously when using a feel-doe vibrator, which can result in violent orgasms while they thrust.

Chapter Five: Focusing on Her Pleasure to Make Her Happy

A Shared Experience

Making female pleasure a priority changes the close relationship into one in which both parties experience joy, connection, and mutual fulfillment. It promotes equality and candid communication by questioning established conventions. As they set out on this journey together, partners learn that the real meaning of intimacy is found in the pursuit of pleasure shared by both parties, weaving a rich and satisfying tapestry of experiences that goes beyond conventional norms.

The Cornerstone of Intimacy: Building a Foundation of Trust and Connection

Setting her pleasure first has a significant impact on the fundamental components of connection and trust, so it's not just about the act itself. Open communication acts as the glue that holds lovers together, shared vulnerability deepens the bond, and trust becomes the cornerstone around which intimacy is constructed. As couples set out on this path of pleasure, they find that building a foundation based on trust, connection, and a shared commitment to each other's happiness is what really defines intimacy.

Trust as the Foundation: Trust serves as the foundation upon which the structure of intimacy is built. Prioritizing her pleasure shows that a partner is committed to knowing and fulfilling her wants, which instills a sense of security in the partnership. This trust penetrates the emotional and psychological spheres in addition to the physical one, creating a basis upon which both partners are free to be honest, transparent, and true to who they are.

A partner who pursues her pleasure shows dependability, constancy, and a sincere interest in the experience together. This steadfast dedication to comprehending and meeting her needs gradually cultivates trust and creates a setting in which both parties feel emotionally secure. Partners who have a deeper level of trust are more sensitive to each other's weaknesses, which strengthens their bond.

Establishing Connection by Mutual Vulnerability: Mutual vulnerability is the foundation of intimacy. Setting her pleasure as a top priority entails exploring the emotional and psychological components that contribute to her fulfillment in addition to her physical desires. Through this mutual exploration of vulnerability, a bond is formed that goes beyond the surface and explores the deepest hopes, anxieties, and wants of each person.

A partner's proactive efforts to comprehend and meet her needs start a reciprocal exchange of vulnerability. Both people participate in a reciprocal disclosure of their deepest selves, which cultivates a close and genuine bond. A deeper and more lasting connection, where partners feel seen, heard, and deeply known, is built on this shared vulnerability.

Open Communication as the Bridge: Open communication is essential to building connections and trust. Setting her pleasure first requires a deeper conversation than just surface-level banter. Conversations concerning desires, limits, and changing preferences are had by partners. Through mutual understanding that goes beyond presumptions or preconceptions, this communication serves as a bridge to link them on a deeper level.

Couples learn to negotiate the nuances of each other's enjoyment through honest conversation. It turns into a tool for communicating needs, investigating desires, and resolving issues. A relationship dynamic where both parties actively participate in co-creating their personal experiences is facilitated by this open communication. The sharing of ideas and aspirations deepens the emotional tie by fostering an intimate sort of connection in and of itself.

The Convergence of Pleasure and Trust: Prioritizing her pleasure and establishing trust and connection has a cascading impact that goes well beyond the intimate times. It seeps into other areas of the partnership, impacting emotional support, communication, and general relationship happiness. When a foundation is based on connection and trust, it stabilizes the relationship throughout difficult times and forges a strong link that endures life's ups and downs.

Breaking Down Social Expectations in Sexual Relationships

Intimate relationship norms can be broken down in a liberating and transformational way. It entails putting gendered narratives to the test, accepting equality in pleasure, encouraging candid conversation, developing an inclusive sexual environment, and establishing a consent-and respect-centered culture. Couples engage on a journey that frees pleasure from predetermined roles and enables a more genuine, varied, and fulfilling intimate relationship by breaking down the limits imposed by society conventions. Her enjoyment becomes a communal endeavor in this emancipated arena, beyond the constraints of conventional expectations and honoring the individuality of every person's needs.

Communication as the Cornerstone:
She needs effective communication to prioritize her pleasure on her trip. It entails having frank conversations about preferences, boundaries, and desires. By establishing a roadmap for exploration, this conversation makes sure that both partners are aware of one another's needs and actively participate in the search of pleasure together. Communication turns into a tool for mutual growth, understanding, and connection.

The gendered narrative surrounding pleasure is frequently woven by societal expectations, which uphold conventional roles that specify who should be the main source of fulfillment. These assumptions have historically placed the onus of delivering pleasure on males, leaving women as passive recipients. To demolish established norms, one must deconstruct this gendered narrative, acknowledge that enjoyment is a shared responsibility, and should not be confined predefined roles.

Couples set out to redefine their responsibilities in the intimate relationship by questioning these standards. By recognizing that both parties actively contribute to a fulfilling sexual encounter, society's constrictive barriers are broken down, promoting a more equal and free attitude toward pleasure.

Accepting Equality in Pleasure: Accepting equality in pleasure is the same as shattering social norms. It denotes a shift from the idea that pleasure is a one-way trip and emphasizes the significance of satisfying both parties. Open communication about needs and desires between partners is encouraged, creating a setting where both parties actively participate in the pursuit of pleasure.

Her enjoyment is the primary focus of the personal experience rather than a secondary consideration in an unbiased approach. This change releases enjoyment from the confines of cultural norms and contradicts deeply held notions about gender roles.

It creates the possibility of a more harmonious and balanced sexual dynamic in which both parties feel free to freely express their wants.

Dispelling Stereotypes Through Open Communication: Transcending social norms can be accomplished with the use of open communication. Partners have deep talks that challenge preconceived notions and stereotypes that are embedded in society standards. Couples can create a space where genuine communication becomes the driving force behind their intimate connection by being transparent about their wishes, boundaries, and dreams.

The preconception that women should be submissive in communicating their needs or that men should naturally comprehend women's enjoyment is dispelled by this conversation. Rather, it encourages a transparent culture in which couples actively participate in co-creating their sexual encounters. By having an honest conversation, partners can unlearn cultural norms and develop a special, welcoming attitude to pleasure.

Creating an Inclusive Sexual environment: The first step in establishing an inclusive sexual environment is dismantling cultural expectations. It entails appreciating and acknowledging the variety of goals, tastes, and ways of expressing them in a partnership. Couples are encouraged to explore their particular preferences and talk freely about what makes them happy, creating a culture that celebrates individuality rather than stifles it.

Her enjoyment in this accepting environment is not limited by preconceived ideas of what is considered appropriate. Without worrying about being judged, couples are able to explore a broad spectrum of preferences, from the traditional to the unusual. This flexibility releases pleasure from the limitations of social norms, enabling partners to create a sexual encounter that speaks to their particular relationship.

Developing a Culture of Consent and Respect: Dismantling social norms naturally promotes a consent and respectful culture. Partners who actively question expectations foster an atmosphere in which limits are acknowledged and spoken for. Beyond the conventional idea that one partner's pleasure comes before the other's, consent becomes an ongoing, joyful exchange.

The emphasis is shifted from presumptions to active communication in this culture of permission and respect. By reaffirming that each partner's comfort and happiness are equally important, it challenges the historical disparity that has been supported by social norms. In order to make sure that pleasure is a shared and consenting experience, partners work together.

Accepting the Diversity of Desire: Accepting the diversity of desire is a life-changing experience that supports the development of a fulfilling and peaceful intimate relationship. In order to successfully negotiate this complex terrain, partners must comprehend the complex nature of desire, communicate openly, embrace individuality, explore novelty and flexibility, and negotiate varying degrees of desire with empathy.

Couples that go out on this path come to realize that the mosaic of many desires they weave together is what makes intimacy beautiful. It's an admission that desire is a dynamic force that calls for understanding, inquiry, and cooperative investigation rather than a static object. Couples who embrace the diversity of desire open the door to a genuinely fulfilling relationship that changes over time to reflect the many details of their shared passion.

Recognizing the Complex Nature of Desire: Intimate relationships involve a variety of complex aspects, including desire in all of its manifestations. It includes a range of inclinations, dreams, and subtle emotional aspects that enhance the depth of the personal encounter. In order to embrace the diversity of want, one must recognize that there is no one-size-fits-all template and that each partner's desires are different and that desire is inherently dynamic.

In this setting, partners are urged to see desire as a dynamic energy that adapts to their own development, outside factors, and shifting situations rather than as a static thing. Understanding the complexity of desire acts as a catalyst for fostering an atmosphere in which partners feel heard, understood, and validated in their own displays of passion.

Managing Communication About Desire: Good communication is essential to embracing the diversity of desire. Couples have frank conversations about their goals, limits, and changing preferences. This communication helps each other develop a profound awareness of each other's deepest goals in addition to being a tool of practical trade.

Couples who communicate openly manage the complexities of desire and develop a mutual language that transcends words. In order to navigate the complex terrain of desire, partners must learn to interpret the nonverbal clues, minute details, and changing requirements. They are profoundly connected to one another through this conversation, which creates an atmosphere in which the depth of desire is acknowledged and explored.

Honoring Individuality in Desire: Every person enters a relationship with a distinct set of desires that have been shaped by their own experiences, cultural influences, and ongoing self-discovery. Rather than aiming for conformity, embracing the diversity of desire entails recognizing this individuality. It is recommended that partners acknowledge and value the uniqueness of one another's wishes, acknowledging that these distinctions add to the complexity of their relationship.

Celebrating the uniqueness of desire challenges the idea that there is a single, widely recognized definition of passion. Rather, it invites couples to savor the abundance that results from the intersection of two distinct sets of desires. The foundation of a relationship dynamic where partners accept and value each other's varied manifestations of passion is laid by this celebration of individuality.

Exploring Novelty and Adaptability: As desire changes throughout time, it is necessary to be open to investigating novelties and adaptabilities. A common commitment to navigate this changing terrain with openness and curiosity is necessary to embrace the diversity of desire. Partners try out new experiences, delve into new aspects of want, and stay flexible in the face of shifting passion dynamics.

Exploring novelty can entail attempting unusual, private pursuits, experimenting with various environments, or adding aspects of surprise. Desire is not limited to routine in this dynamic atmosphere created by this openness to adapt; rather, it flourishes on the thrill of shared discovery. It supports the notion that the discovery of desire is a continuous process in which both partners actively participate in its development.

Handling Various Desire Levels: Throughout the course of an intimate relationship, partners may feel varying degrees of desire. Managing these swings with compassion, comprehension, and clear communication is part of accepting the diversity of desire. Couples address these variations with a sense of shared responsibility, understanding that stress, health, and life events can all have an impact on desire.

It takes a dedication to mutual support and a readiness to adjust to each other's needs to navigate various levels of desire. Couples converse about differences in desire without passing judgment on one another, creating a space where each person feels understood and encouraged. This navigation turns into a cooperative endeavor to uphold a harmonious equilibrium that takes into account the dynamic character of desire.

The Power of Reciprocity: Giving her joy priority is a two-way street. It entails the reciprocal trade of fulfillment and desire. Partners can initiate a positive cycle of reciprocity in which both parties actively contribute to each other's satisfaction by concentrating on her pleasure. This reciprocal commitment strengthens the bond and guarantees that intimacy is a joyful and fulfilling journey that is experienced by both parties.

Enhancing Emotional Connection: In an intimate relationship, mutual enjoyment plays a role in enhancing emotional connection. It creates a sense of intimacy that goes beyond social conventions and extends beyond the physical act. Partners learn to read each other's reactions, resulting in a harmonious pleasure-giving exchange that strengthens the emotional connection. Making her pleasure a priority opens the door to a deeper and more fulfilling relationship.

Quality Above Quantity: Placing her enjoyment first causes the emphasis to change from quantity to quality. The depth and fulfillment that each personal experience brings is what matters, not how often you have them. Couples learn to live in the now and approach sensuality with greater awareness and purpose. This focus on quality makes sure that the experiences that are shared are rewarding and unforgettable.

Long-Term partnership Satisfaction: Setting her pleasure as a top priority in a long-term partnership becomes a sustaining factor. It enhances the relationship's stability and general level of satisfaction. Couples' dedication to enjoying each other's company throughout their journey together guarantees that their relationship will always be lively, thrilling, and incredibly satisfying.

Empowering Both parties: In a close relationship, putting her pleasure first strengthens both parties. It promotes a sense of shared action and equality by dispelling the myth that one partner is exclusively responsible for one's pleasure. Prioritizing her pleasure gives her the empowerment she needs to establish an environment where both of them feel free to express their wishes and actively contribute to each other's joy.

Exploring Desire: A Shared Path to Satisfaction

Intimate partnerships undergo a transforming journey when partners are encouraged to explore each other's interests and actively contribute to a shared, fulfilling experience. It entails the capacity to comprehend desires, establish an atmosphere of candid communication, traverse unfamiliar ground, participate in the reciprocal act of contributing, and promote a shared growth culture.

The Power of Understanding Desires: A deeper level of connection can be established by having an understanding of one another's desires. It entails exploring the subtleties of what makes each partner feel happy, satisfied, and intimate. Partners can explore the complexities of desire together and develop a deeper connection by deliberately seeking to understand one other better. This can be achieved by providing a path for their shared discovery.

Partners get insight into the emotional, psychological, and physical aspects that go into satisfaction when they are aware of each other's needs. This knowledge turns into a powerful tool for building empathy and a space where each person feels appreciated and seen for the distinctive ways they express their enthusiasm.

Establishing an Environment of Open Communication: Open communication is essential to promoting the exploration of wishes. Couples have open and sincere conversations about their desires, whims, and changing needs. This conversation is more than just a business deal; it's a deep exchange of weaknesses, hopes, and the subtleties of what makes us passionate.

Open communication allows partners to freely express their preferences without worrying about being judged. It turns into a place where desires are expressed, boundaries are discussed, and fantasies are revealed. When partners actively participate in co-creating their personal encounters, this openness serves as the foundation for a relationship dynamic.

Finding Your Way Through unexplored Desire area: It is implied that exploring wants requires a willingness to go through unexplored area. It entails venturing beyond one's comfort zone, welcoming change, and partaking in activities together that enhance the depth of the personal journey. Together, partners explore each other's imaginations, try out various pastimes, and create an atmosphere that is enhanced by the thrill of the unknown.

To successfully navigate the unexplored region of wishes, one must be open-minded and curious. It entails a common dedication to broadening the scope of enjoyment, incorporating aspects of surprise, and creating an atmosphere where discovery turns into a fun and exciting activity. Along the way, couples learn that the unexplored world of desires is a blank canvas on which they can paint the bright colors of their desires.

Promoting couples to investigate their aspirations is a mutually beneficial undertaking that involves both parties contributing in some way. By carefully listening to and satisfying each other's needs, the two people establish a constructive cycle of reciprocity. This shared commitment acts as a spark to strengthen the bond and guarantee that the intimate experience is a joyful and fulfilling journey for both parties.

Understanding and actively contributing to the fulfillment of desires are both components of the reciprocal act of contribution. Partners learn to interpret each other's reactions and tiny indications that indicate contentment, becoming more attuned to one another's replies. With both parties actively participating in the creation of moments of deep connection, the intimate experience becomes a dance of shared passion.

Promoting a Culture of Shared Growth:
Encouraging an exploration of desires goes beyond the here and now and instead cultivates a culture of

shared growth in the partnership. As partners actively support one another's happiness, they set out on a path of individual and group growth. This mutual development turns into a proof of the relationship's flexibility and the changing nature of desire.

It's important to acknowledge that desires change with time in order to promote a culture of shared progress. It calls for partners to embrace the dynamic nature of their relationship, adjust to shifting tastes, and discover new pleasures. The encouragement to follow one's desires in this culture translates into a lifetime dedication to mutual fulfillment, understanding, and the ongoing development of the close relationship.

Chapter Six: Embracing Confidence and Fostering Positive Body Image

A Journey of Self-Love

Developing a positive body image and embracing confidence are transformative journeys that lead to self-discovery, empowerment, and emancipation. It entails comprehending the intricacies of one's own self-perception, resisting social pressures, embracing the deep core of self-acceptance and love, and empowering techniques for boosting self-esteem and good body image.

People that go on this powerful journey come to realize that genuine beauty comes from the inside out and is shown through self-love, confidence, and sincerity. It is a journey that surpasses standards set by society, frees people from the grip of perfectionism, and honors the individuality and beauty that each person possesses.

Recognizing the Complicated Terrain of Self-Perception: Personal experiences, societal conventions, and cultural values all influence how one perceives oneself. This is due to the complex interaction of internal and external influences. Self-confidence and body image issues are frequently the result of the complex dance that goes on between our own viewpoints and the norms that are ingrained in society.

Individuals' perceptions of themselves are greatly influenced by internal factors such as upbringing, experiences, and innate self-worth. Conversely, external elements consist of cultural norms, media representations, and societal expectations that establish standards for acceptable beauty and behavior. A sophisticated grasp of these factors and a deliberate attempt to separate one's own value from opinions of others are necessary for navigating this challenging terrain.

Societal Influences' Effect on Body Image
The effects of cultural influences on body image traverse a challenging landscape of socially manufactured ideals, coercive conformity, and the fallout from defying expectations. For those attempting to develop a positive and genuine body image, it is imperative to comprehend the ubiquitous nature of these impacts.

There is a chance for empowerment, resistance, and reinvention as society struggles with changing ideas of beauty. Promoting media literacy, strengthening resistance against unattainable standards, accepting variety, and questioning conventional wisdom are all steps in the process of cultivating a good body image. People learn how to construct their own narratives, set their own standards of beauty, and set out on a life-changing path of self-acceptance and empowerment through this complex exploration.

The All-Pervasiveness of Social Standards: From the glossy pages of magazines to the digital spaces of social media, societal standards of beauty are present in every aspect of contemporary life. These criteria produce an omnipresent narrative that sets limited conceptions of attractiveness. They are frequently determined by fashion trends, media depictions, and prevalent cultural norms. People who traverse this terrain will unavoidably come across pictures and messaging that establish standards for physical beauty and shape their ideas of an idealized self.

In media portrayals, where airbrushed photos and carefully chosen representations reinforce an exaggerated and homogenized idea of beauty, the pervasiveness of societal norms is especially clear. Because of this widespread exposure, these ideals become internalized by the general public, which affects how people view their own bodies and, in turn, their self-worth.

Building Beauty Ideals: Social factors are crucial in the creation and maintenance of beauty ideals, which frequently marginalize diversity and elevate a limited range of physical characteristics as attractive. People's ideas of what is deemed acceptable or attractive are influenced by these values, whether they are actively acknowledged or unconsciously assimilated.

Beauty standards are not created in a vacuum; historical, cultural, and economic influences all have a role. For instance, historically ingrained and still prevalent in many countries, Eurocentric beauty standards exclude and diminish the beauty of those who defy them. Determining how these standards affect body image and promoting an open and tolerant viewpoint require an understanding of how these ideals are produced.

The Struggle for Conformity: People frequently struggle with a pervasive sense of inadequacy and the pressure to achieve an impossible ideal in their effort to conform to society beauty standards. The pursuit of conformity can take many different forms; it might involve rigorous exercise routines and restrictive eating plans, as well as cosmetic surgery in an effort to meet social norms.

The quest for conformity turns into a precarious balancing act where people risk becoming caught up in a vicious cycle of self-criticism, comparison, and discontent. The constant search for an unattainable ideal can be demoralizing and lead to a widespread belief that one does not live up to the socially acceptable standards of beauty.

The negative effects of non-conformity, which frequently take the form of body shaming and stigmatization, can befall people who don't conform to society's standards of beauty. It is possible for those who question conventional notions of beauty to face social alienation, prejudice, and judgment, which increases the need to fit in.

Body shaming can have significant psychological and emotional effects and is often driven by societal forces. It could have a role in the emergence of poor self-esteem, negative body image, and mental health issues. A cycle of shame and insecurity is maintained by the stigma attached to nonconformity, which encourages people to hide, change, or apologize for their bodies.

Embracing Resistance and Redefining Beauty:
There is a growing movement of empowerment and resistance in spite of the pervasive influence of societal pressures on body image. People and groups are questioning conventional wisdom, promoting tolerance, and redefining beauty according to their own standards.

Deconstructing the stereotypes of beauty that are spread by society is a necessary step in empowering resistance. It inspires people to reject homogeneity in conventional beauty standards and embrace variation and individuality. Social media platforms have developed into effective tools that people can use to highlight a variety of body types, promoting a feeling of community and legitimizing portrayals that go against accepted norms.

Promoting Media Literacy and Critical Awareness:
Promoting media literacy and critical awareness is essential to addressing how society influences body image. People are able to actively participate in analyzing and challenging the pictures and ideas that the media presents. Having a perceptive eye enables people to identify the frequently distorted and idealized portrayals that support unattainable beauty standards.

People who receive media literacy training are better equipped to analyze the manufactured nature of beauty standards, recognize the impact of business interests, and gain more discernment when it comes to the images they see. This critical consciousness serves as a defense against the detrimental effects of internalizing unreachable ideals of beauty.

Developing Self-Worth and Body Positivity: Empowering Techniques for Increasing Confidence Regardless of Body Size

In an environment where cultural norms frequently uphold limited conceptions of beauty, developing self-confidence—particularly with regard to body size—becomes a complex and empowering process. This essay examines methods that people of all body sizes can use to develop confidence, with a focus on physical well-being, positive self-talk, inclusion in fashion, self-acceptance, and the importance of a supportive community. By challenging social standards and adopting a holistic perspective, people can start down a transformative journey toward self-assurance and body positivity.

Embracing Self-Acceptance Beyond Societal Norms: This is the first step towards developing confidence. It involves accepting who you are in spite of social conventions. People gain from appreciating and celebrating the intrinsic value of their bodies, regardless of size. This entails tearing down preconceived conceptions of beauty imposed by outside norms and realizing that genuine confidence arises from accepting one's distinct physical characteristics.

The path to self-acceptance involves changing the way one talks to oneself and adopting an outlook that values beauty in all of its manifestations. Through questioning cultural conventions that uphold unattainable body standards, people can free themselves from the bonds of conformity and establish a foundation for developing authentically confident confidence.

Affirmations & Positive Self-Talk for Body Positivity:
Affirmations and constructive self-talk are essential for boosting confidence, particularly with regard to body image. People can deliberately create a conversation that supports self-love and body positivity. This entails using affirmations that

highlight the body's strength, adaptability, and distinctive qualities to overcome negative beliefs.

Body positive affirmations help rewire internal narratives and cultivate an appreciation of oneself that surpasses social criticism. People can change the way they perceive themselves and develop confidence that is unaffected by other people's opinions by continuously receiving good messages about their bodies.

Placing Physical Health Above Conformity: Prioritizing one's physical health over meeting social norms is a key component of body-positive building. This method places a strong emphasis on leading a healthy lifestyle that enhances general wellbeing regardless of social norms. Regular exercise and mindful eating are two examples of physical health-promoting behaviors that can be used as a tool for self-care and self-empowerment.

People change the narrative from reaching a specific body size to taking care of their bodies for optimal health when they place more emphasis on physical well-being. This holistic viewpoint highlights the link between mental and physical health, supporting the development of a positive self-concept and self-assurance that result from a sense of empowerment and self-care.

Building Confidence and Fostering Positive Self-Perception in the Context of Sexual Satisfaction

In the context of sexual fulfillment, developing self-worth and positive self-perception requires an all-encompassing process that incorporates self-analysis, candid dialogue, body positivity, discovery, and the strength of understanding one another. This comprehensive approach emphasizes the value of both individual and mutual well-being in intimate relationships, going beyond what is typically expected of it.

People who go on this life-changing adventure learn that having sex is more than just a physical act; it's a deep and complex investigation of desires, feelings, and understanding between people. Confidence and a strong self-image combined weave a fabric that takes personal experiences to a new level of fulfillment that celebrates the individuality of every person and the strength of emotional connection in the complexities of sexual fulfillment.

Self-Evaluation as the Basis:
Self-reflection is the first step on the path to developing positive self-perception and sexual confidence. People gain from self-examination that explores boundaries, personal desires, and the elements that influence a sense of sexual self-worth in addition to physical characteristics. This process entails appreciating and embracing one's individuality, figuring out what makes one happy, and realizing how closely physical and emotional health are related.

People make room for a deeper awareness of their own preferences, comfort zones, and desires through self-reflection. Because it synchronizes personal ideals with intimate experiences and cultivates a positive self-perception that goes beyond social standards, this awareness serves as a basis for the development of sexual confidence.

Open Communication and Mutual Understanding:
When it comes to sexual happiness, communication is essential. It helps to develop good self-perception and boost self-confidence. With a relationship, open and honest communication creates a space in which expectations, boundaries, and wants may all be freely shared and understood. Through this reciprocal communication, a climate of trust is

created, which helps to eliminate fears and build confidence based on shared knowledge.

Active listening, empathy, and a readiness to discuss desires and worries are all necessary for effective communication. Open and honest communication between partners not only lays the groundwork for fulfilling encounters, but it also affirms and respects each other's positive self-perceptions.

Adopting Body Positivity and Self-Love: Developing body positivity and self-love has a profoundly transformational effect on one's sexual self-perception and confidence. In a culture where limited beauty standards frequently impact people, people may bring insecurities into personal relationships. Choosing to celebrate the body's special qualities and skills rather than focusing on perceived defects is a key component of embracing body positivity.

Self-affirmations, appreciating the beauty of all body shapes, and partaking in self-care routines that cultivate a good relationship with one's own body are among the practices that support body positivity. When people are confident in their body and embrace self-love, it fosters an environment where both partners may enjoy and respect each other's bodies without bias or unreasonable expectations.

Exploration and Playful Curiosity in Close Relationships: In close relationships, exploration and playful curiosity create a fabric of mutual joy, connection, and discovery. Couples who embrace adventure set out on a trip that goes beyond the physical and explores the emotional and psychological spheres. Open communication, vulnerability, trust, and a fun attitude foster an environment where intimacy is explored in a dynamic and ever-changing way.

The Purpose of Exploration: Intimate relationship exploration goes beyond the ordinary and customary, beckoning people and their partners to explore previously unexplored emotional depths, dreams, and desires.
It entails taking an intentional and receptive approach to learning about new aspects of oneself and one's spouse. Physical, emotional, and psychological domains are all included in exploration, which creates a dynamic environment where limits are gently challenged and vulnerabilities are welcomed.

Finding new pleasure zones and sensual nuances are all part of the physical exploration process. Together, partners embark on a journey to comprehend each other's bodies, preferences, and reactions. This process creates an atmosphere in which mutual discoveries serve as a source of fulfillment and connection.

Understanding one other's complex emotions, anxieties, and goals is achieved through emotional inquiry. Emotional vulnerabilities are recognized and valued in a space created by partners having candid and open discussions. This degree of investigation builds a foundation for a strong and emotionally close relationship by fostering a deeper understanding and connection.

Partners are invited to peel back the layers of each other's wants, imaginations, and mental landscapes through psychological investigation. This includes role-playing, discussing psychological subtleties that enhance the depth of the intimate relationship, and jointly exploring fantasies.

Playful Curiosity as the Catalyst: Playful curiosity is the catalyst that drives discovery. Playful curiosity creates an environment where partners feel free to express themselves honestly by bringing a sense of lightheartedness and joy to the process of discovery. It entails taking an adventurous, open-minded, and welcoming attitude toward the unexpected when it comes to intimate exploration.

The delight of joint discovery is the fuel of playful curiosity. Playfully setting off on exploratory adventures, partners foster an atmosphere where spontaneity and experimentation are essential elements of the close relationship. This kind of thinking goes beyond stereotypes and enables people and partners to partake in enjoyable activities that promote joy, laughter, and a rekindled sense of connection.

Curiosity's playful quality allows partners to see intimate exploration as a continuous and changing process. It encourages an attitude that values making mistakes, communicates freely, and places more emphasis on the delight of joint learning than on perfection. This playful approach helps create a happy, lively environment where couples can express themselves without worrying about being judged.

Traveling Through New Territories: Partners frequently travel through new emotional and physical landscapes as a result of exploration and lighthearted curiosity. This entails embracing an adventurous mindset, venturing beyond of comfort zones, and attempting new things. Exploring new ground becomes a joint effort, whether it's trying out new intimate techniques, adding fresh components to the partnership, or participating in thrilling activities together.

Physically, discovering new erogenous zones, experimenting with sensory sensations, or trying out various forms of physical intimacy can all be part of traversing new territory. Addressing difficult subjects, displaying vulnerability, and strengthening the emotional bond are some examples of emotional navigation. Collectively, these exploratory endeavors support a feeling of resilience and growth among all parties.

Effective communication acts as the compass that leads partners through the world of discovery and fun curiosity. Clear communication of expectations, boundaries, and wishes is made possible by open and honest conversation. By being open and honest, it creates a trusting atmosphere that enables partners to negotiate the subtleties of exploration with mutual understanding.

Actively listening to one another's needs, offering criticism, and expressing comfort levels are all parts of communication. Couples have constant dialogues that change as the exploring process progresses. Both parties will feel heard, appreciated, and empowered to voice their needs and desires thanks to this dynamic conversation.

The Significance of Vulnerability and Trust:
An environment of vulnerability and trust fosters exploration and joyful curiosity. Couples can feel comfortable expressing their wishes because they know that their vulnerabilities will be understood and accepted. This is made possible by trust. When there is this degree of confidence, partners can explore new areas together in safety and without worrying about being judged.

When it comes to personal exploration, vulnerability becomes a potent tool that lets partners honestly communicate their desires and anxieties. People who embrace vulnerability strengthen their emotional bonds and foster a sense of closeness that transcends the physical. Vulnerability between partners is reciprocated, and this serves as a fuel for mutual growth and relationship strengthening.

The Power of Emotional Connection and Mutual Understanding: It is impossible to overestimate the importance of emotional connection and mutual understanding in the context of sexual enjoyment. Developing a sense of safety and trust with a partner is closely related to feeling emotionally connected to them. People who experience emotional intimacy report feeling better about themselves because they have a stronger bond that goes beyond physical proximity.

Understanding one another's emotional needs entails fostering a culture in which being vulnerable is valued and accepted. Mutual understanding creates an emotional bond that grows stronger and serves as a basis for the development of sexual confidence. People's good self-perceptions flow into their personal experiences when they feel recognized, appreciated, and emotionally linked. This creates a harmonious and satisfying connection.

Conclusion

Taking Pleasure Above and Beyond Size

The book "Great Sex! Over Size" acts as a compass on the path to amazing and satisfying sex encounters by guiding readers through the treacherous territory of close relationships through an open examination of sex secrets. By the time we finish this insightful investigation, it will be clear that the main idea is to take pleasure beyond the realm of the physical. The focus on incredible, thrilling, and sensational sex practices becomes evidence of the transformational potential that results from placing skills and communication above the obsessions that society has with size.

Recap of Key Insights:

The handbook challenges traditional ideas about sexual fulfillment by weaving together a number of important insights. By exposing the fallacy that enjoyment is solely determined by size, it undermines social constraints and promotes a more inclusive narrative. The voyage reveals that the key to a genuinely fulfilling intimate relationship is the investigation of sexual techniques, communication, and the celebration of various desires.

The story highlights the holistic nature of sexual fulfillment and how it is closely related to emotional connection, communication, and the openness to experience new kinds of pleasure. It breaks down preconceptions and inspires people to accept their own aspirations and expressions, cultivating an attitude that values the variety of close relationships.

Prioritizing Techniques Over Size: This guide's central concept is the importance of giving techniques precedence over size. It contradicts the widely accepted societal narrative that associates pleasure only with physical attributes. The guide enables people to concentrate on the artistry of intimacy by highlighting particular sex techniques and unfiltered secrets. It emphasizes that technique mastery plays a large role in satisfaction, regardless of size.

By shifting the emphasis from outside forces to the interior dynamics of relationships, this main topic acts as a paradigm shift. It promotes an attitude that values the distinctive features of every person and creates an atmosphere in which couples may interact, explore, and adapt together.

The guidance acts as a lighthouse at the end, encouraging people and partners to adopt a mindset of constant research, communication, and adaptation. Curiosity, candid communication, and flexibility are portrayed as the guiding principles of an ongoing inquiry that leads to extraordinary and fulfilling sexual partnerships.

Constant exploration creates an environment of freshness and excitement by requiring people to be open to discovering and rediscovering one other's desires. When partners are able to share their wants, boundaries, and fantasies without fear of being judged, open communication becomes the cornerstone. The dynamic force that permits relationships to change and guarantees that intimacy stays a lively and fulfilling part of the partnership is adaptation, as the handbook encourages.

"Great Sex! Over Size" appears as a paradigm shift in how we view and treat intimate relationships, not just as a manual. It dispels preconceived notions, gives people the confidence to value methods over size, and promotes an attitude of constant inquiry, dialogue, and adaptability. Equipped with unfiltered sex secrets, readers are challenged to adopt a holistic perspective that embraces the rich shades of human closeness and elevates pleasure beyond social limits as they set out on their journeys toward meaningful sexual relationships.

www.ingramcontent.com/pod-product-compliance
Lightning Source LLC
Chambersburg PA
CBHW070951260726
48661CB00003B/1228